Ketogenic Diet For Beginners

———— ❧❧❧ ————

A Simplified Perspective About Ketosis With Amazing Weight Loss Recipes

By Jennifer Sullivan

Free Gift

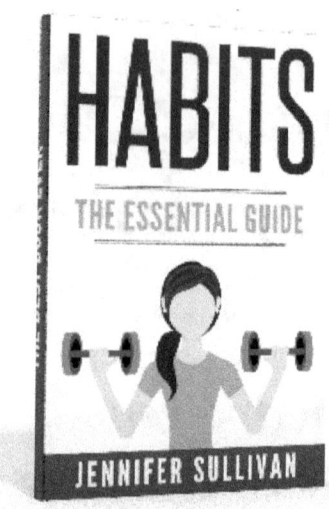

Discover The Secrets Behind How You Can Hardwire Your Brain For Success With Simple Habits!

Smoking, skipping breakfast, and procrastinating, these are some of the habits that we all know we should change and erase from our lives. However, even if changing these habits have been a part of your resolution list for so many New Years', it's still hard to let these habits go. Well, let me tell you that it is going to change now.

Not Everyone Wants To Admit It

To become the best you, you must stop looking at the big picture and start working on the small yet important stuff—your habits!

>>Visit This Link To Download "Habits: The Essential Guide" For FREE<<

https://cueballpublishing.leadpages.co/ free-habits-ebook/

Introduction

I want to thank you and congratulate you for purchasing my book, *"Ketogenic Diet For Beginners: A Simplified Perspective About Ketosis With Amazing Weight Loss Recipes"*.

This book focuses on the strong foundations of the ketogenic diet to grant you confidence in your journey to a happier and more vibrant lifestyle!

A good diet shouldn't be a transitory chore, but a gateway to sustainable, life-long improvements. It should allow you to build the energy and positivity you need to maintain a healthy body weight, manage any health conditions and boost your zest for living. The ketogenic diet means just that - an easy, medically supported eating plan that restricts your carbs without restricting your possibilities.

Reaching your long-term lifestyle goals can be challenging, especially if you're not enjoying the journey there. But building motivation becomes a lot easier when you're eating quick and easy, delicious foods that you've prepared yourself.

Thanks again for joining me. Enjoy!

The information herein is offered for informational purposes solely, and is universal as so. The presentation of the information is without contract or any type of guarantee assurance.

The trademarks that are used are without any consent, and the publication of the trademark is without permission or backing by the trademark owner. All trademarks and brands within this book are for clarifying purposes only and are the owned by the owners themselves, not affiliated with this document.

Table of Contents

What is the ketogenic diet?

The fancy sounding term 'ketogenic diet' can be a bit intimidating at first. But what it describes is simply a low carb, high fat eating regime that forces the body to use fats for energy rather than carbohydrates. In a traditional diet, the carbs obtained from food are broken down into their simplest form - glucose, which is then transported via the blood stream to all the organs in the body.

One particular organ - the brain - is especially demanding, drawing over 20% of all the glucose circulating the blood stream. However, if there aren't enough carbs available in one's diet, the body enters a special metabolic state in which the liver converts fat into fatty acids and ketone bodies. This metabolic state is called *ketosis*, and it also manifests during prolonged fasting periods.

When ketosis is achieved, ketone bodies simply replace glucose as the main source of energy for the brain and every other organ. The ketogenic diet is somewhat similar to the low-carb and Atkins diets, but it differs in that it has more specific guidelines, and the primary goal of inducing ketosis.

How does ketosis improve health?

Since ancient times, periods of extended fasting have been hailed for their rejuvenating and curative properties. The modern version of the ketogenic diet emerged in the 1920s, when doctors tested its therapeutic benefits in controlling epilepsy in children.

Since then, it has proven useful in treating a myriad of other conditions, including type 2 diabetes, autism, depression, polycystic ovary syndrome, and a range of neurodegenerative disorders such as ALS, Alzheimer's and Parkinson's.

A 2014 medical review showed that ketosis might be helpful in supporting traditional cancer treatments. Since tumor cells rely specifically on glucose metabolism to thrive, they are ineffective at processing ketone bodies. Several studies conducted over the last 25 years have found that ketogenic regimes improve survival and reduce tumor growth in malignant glioma, colon cancer, gastric cancer, lung cancer and prostate cancer.

A quality of life study found no adverse effects in cancer patients on a ketogenic diet, while other studies suggest ketosis may improve radiation and chemotherapy response and reduce the severity of any adverse effects.

More recent evidence suggests it may even be protective against traumatic brain injury and may help with stroke recovery.

Why you should cut back on carbs

An old dieting myth that just won't go away attributes weight gain to fat consumption, but in reality, things are less intuitive: the new fat that our bodies store is derived primarily from carbs. Simply put, fat doesn't make you fat, sugar and bread do. During ketosis, fat isn't stored, it is used for energy. This is an ideal situation if your goal is weight loss, because it encourages the liver to tap into already stored fat reserves.

Carbs are also responsible for elevated blood sugar levels, which can lead to diabetes. This makes the ketogenic diet an optimal regime for glycemic control and improved insulin sensitivity.

The relationship between the carbs consumed and the insulin produced is directly proportional, meaning that the more carbohydrates you consume, the more insulin your body is forced to produce in an attempt to control them. Sadly, insulin is also a fat storing hormone, so if your body is encouraged to produce more, it will make shedding off unwanted weight very difficult.

If you've been wondering why you have a hard time dropping extra pounds even though you're seemingly eating all the right foods, this might just be your answer.

Going keto is beginner-friendly

Are you worried that your cooking skills might not be up to snuff or that you won't be able to find some obscure, exotic ingredients? Don't be! The ketogenic diet is not a fad, it is supported by a wealth of medical evidence, and it is designed to be manageable in the long term. It relies on familiar ingredients and techniques, allowing you to both reconstruct traditional recipes and to get your creative groove on.

Hearty cream soups, sumptuous burgers, yummy pizzas and buttery desserts can be fast and easy to prepare. It draws influence from the Mediterranean and oriental cuisines, so even though it drastically restricts your carb intake, the ketogenic diet doesn't feel restrictive.

You will not have to starve yourself with unsatisfying foods, you still get to eat the foods you like, except now they'll have a deliciously full-fat, low-carb twist!

Keto essentials: what to eat and what to avoid

As we've seen, the main goal of the ketogenic diet is to get your body to primarily use fats for energy, whilst providing adequate levels of protein and other essential nutrients. Let's now take a quick look at the basic guidelines underpinning this diet:

What you shouldn't eat

- All grains, even whole meal (wheat, corn, oats, rye, buckwheat, quinoa, rice) and grain products such as pasta, bread, breakfast cereals

- Potatoes and starchy foods

- Sugar and all sugary products: table sugar, honey, agave syrup, high-fructose corn syrup, non-keto cakes and all other traditional desserts, soft drinks

- All processed foods - trans-fats (hydrogenated oils, margarine, snack foods), artificial sweeteners (aspartame, Acesulfame, sucralose) and processed meat (cold meats, salami and sausages). Unfortunately, although they are high in protein and fat, most commercially processed meats are loaded with chemical additives, making them unhealthy choices

- Some high-sugar tropical fruits (banana, papaya, pineapple) and high-sugar dried fruits (dates, raisins, figs)

What you can eat, but only in moderation

- Legumes - beans, peas, lentils, soybeans and peanuts. These foods are a good source of protein, but they are fairly high in carbs so consider this trade-off when incorporating them in your diet

- Nuts and seeds - they are very nutritious but are packed with calories. A handful is more than enough for 1 serving

- Homemade keto desserts. They will add some carbs to your diet, but within acceptable levels if consumed in moderation

- Natural sugar substitutes - stevia and splenda

What you should eat

- All types of unprocessed meat, fish and eggs - poultry, beef, lamb, turkey, rabbit, wild game, as well as salmon, ocean fish and seafood, including roe

- Healthy fats - saturated: animal fat, butter, ghee, coconut oil

- Monounsaturated: avocado, olive oil, macadamia oil

- Polyunsaturated omega-3 and omega-6: fish oil, canola oil

- Full fat dairy products - yogurt, cheese, heavy cream

- Non-starchy vegetables - leafy greens, cruciferous vegetables and root vegetables (zucchini, asparagus, spinach, lettuce, bok choy, radishes, carrots, celeriac, peppers, onions)

Keto essentials: what to eat and what to avoid

- Most fresh fruits, especially berries - blackberries, blueberries, apples, oranges, cantaloupe

What to drink

- Water - make sure you drink at least 8 tall glasses every day

- Coffee and tea

What you can drink in moderation

- Milk - it is difficult to digest and relatively high in carbs compared to other dairy products, so it's best consumed in small quantities

- Home made almond milk (avoid commercially available versions as they are full of chemical additives)

- Dry wine, with no additives

What beverages to avoid

- Alcoholic drinks high in carbs - cocktails, long drinks, beer

- Fruit juices - while they appear healthy at first glance, keep in mind that they are high in sugar and stripped of all the nutritious fibers you can otherwise find in whole fruits

Benefits of the Ketogenic Diet

There is a lot of negativity that surrounds the ketogenic diet. However, the benefits that one gains from the diet trump the negativity. The benefit that appeals to the masses out there is weight loss since you will lose weight without having to put too much effort since you have started to cut down on the carbohydrate intake. Let us take a look at a few benefits of this diet.

Reduced appetite

On account of the reduced amount of carbohydrates consumed, your body will begin to use the unwanted fat that is in your body to provide your body with enough energy. On many other diets, you tend to starve yourself and will often binge on food that only hinders your weight loss goals.

This diet has the perfect proportions of fats and proteins that make up for the lower carbohydrate content in the food. You will find that your appetite has decreased and that you are able to satiate your hunger.

Loss of abdominal fat

One of the best ways to lose fat in your body would be through some form of exercise. You have to remember that the muscles in your body are very different from each other as is the fat that is stored in the muscles. Some stored fats are more harmful than others and abdominal fat or the visceral fat is extremely harmful.

The fat in this area would start surrounding the organs in the same region thereby hampering their working.

Too much visceral fat in the body causes inflammation, which reduces the insulin that is produced in the body. There are many other health issues that could crop up if you do not control the amount of fat that is in the abdominal region. When you are on the ketogenic diet, the fat in your body is used faster which would help to reduce the fat in the abdomen since you will be consuming fewer carbohydrates.

Weight Loss

When on a diet, people often forget to take into account the carbohydrates that they consume in every meal. A ketogenic diet is a low carbohydrate diet that would assist in the weight loss process.

When you consume fewer carbohydrates, the water that is in excess, in your body will be shed thereby reducing the levels of insulin in your body, which would directly impact the levels of sodium in your body inducing weight loss. Research has confirmed that a low carbohydrate diet will help a person lose weight faster than many other diets.

Lower Blood Pressure

Studies have shown that lower carbohydrate consumption reduces the risk of high blood pressure. This reduces the probability of procuring any heart diseases or other health issues that could prove to be detrimental for your body.

Lower Blood Sugar Levels

The ketogenic diet helps to reduce the level of insulin in the blood thereby reducing the risk of procuring Type II Diabetes.

When you consume carbohydrates, your body breaks them down into sugar components that are then released into the digestive tract. Glucose is one of the main sugar components released into the tract. These components then flow into the bloodstream, which creates an imbalance in the blood sugar levels.

When an imbalance is created, insulin is released to identify which sugar components need to be stored and which are needed to produce energy. If you are healthy, your body will be able to control the release of insulin and prevent Type II Diabetes.

A number of people do suffer from Type II Diabetes. Their body produces too much insulin which causes the body to start resisting or rejecting the insulin produced after a certain threshold. This makes it exceedingly difficult for your body to control the glucose that enters the blood stream thereby increasing the chances of Diabetes, which will cause your body to stop responding to insulin.

The only way to control this is by controlling the number of carbohydrates you consume every meal.

Reducing the Risk of Heart Diseases

When you do not consume food for a long time, your body will produce triglycerides. These compounds are often produced when your body is in the fasting state. When you consume too many carbohydrates in your meals, you will find that you have more triglycerides in your body when compared to someone who consumes fewer carbohydrates.

Triglycerides are a key contributor to heart diseases and it is for this reason that one must reduce the carbohydrate content in their food.

Curing the Metabolic Syndrome

Most people tend to have the metabolic syndrome and would be blind to it. If you have any of the symptoms mentioned below, it would be best if you moved onto a low carbohydrate diet.

1. High Levels of Blood Sugar

2. Low levels of HDL

3. Excess Visceral Fat

4. Hypertension or high blood pressure

5. High levels of Triglycerides

A ketogenic diet helps in reducing the symptoms mentioned thereby reducing the risk of heart diseases and diabetes.

There are certain organizations that have stated that low fat diets are better when compared to low carbohydrate diets since they cater to any metabolic issues that you may have. However, tons of research conducted on the ketogenic diet says otherwise!

Therapeutic for Brain Disorders

It is claimed that glucose is necessary for the brain to function well and this is true. There are some parts of the brain that have the ability to burn glucose while there are other parts of the brain that work towards burning ketones which are formed when the carbohydrate content in the food is low.

This is the mechanism of the ketogenic diet, which was used as therapy to treat children with epilepsy. It was found that this diet worked better than the drugs that the children were asked to use. This diet can be used to cure epilepsy in children and there are studies that show that the seizures due to epilepsy reduce by 50%and close to 15% of the children were free from seizures.

The diet is now being used to see how it can cure or curb the effects of other brain disorders as well.

Setting yourself up for success: 10 tips to boost your motivation

Sometimes it is hard to stick to a new eating regime even if you enjoy it and know that it's good for you. We're constantly bombarded with unhealthy foodstuffs at every street food stall, supermarket and restaurant, and the accessibility of these items makes them hard to pass up.

But before you start beating yourself up over that cheeseburger you had for lunch, remember that changing your eating habits is a long term process, it takes a lot of adjustment and it is not a competition. You cannot really fail at reshaping your diet because every day provides a new opportunity for improvement.

1. *Make incremental changes*

    A common mistake we do when trying to lose weight is to jump right into a new eating routine that is dramatically different from what we are used to eating. While that may work in the short term, it's rarely sustainable and it can sometimes even cause serious health problems because it's such a shock for your body.

    Give yourself time to ease into the keto lifestyle by making small but meaningful changes, like giving up one carb source every couple of weeks. It's important to make sure you've given yourself ample time to adjust to the change before changing anything else. A good way to reduce transition discomfort is to add a healthy nutrient source into your diet every time you take something unhealthy out.

For example, if you've decided to eliminate white flour from your diet, start replacing it with almond flour or coconut flour. This means you can continue to eat biscuits, cookies and even bread on a ketogenic diet.

2. ***Don't give up your favorite foods, turn them keto!***

Thinking of any diet in terms of what you're **not** allowed to eat can quickly become frustrating and discouraging. Instead, look to keto cookbooks and the very inventive keto Internet community for tips and ideas on how to turn traditional dishes into delicious keto-friendly versions.

Keep in mind that going keto is not about deprivation, but about improving your diet and supporting ketosis. Because this is a high fat eating routine, you're still preserving all the deliciousness and texture of your favorite foods. In many cases, the ketogenic diet will even allow you to enhance the flavor of classic dishes by adding luscious ingredients that you might have otherwise shunned, such as heavy cream and melted butter.

3. ***Surround yourself with positivity***

Committing to such a life-changing journey can, at times, be stressing and overwhelming. While it's normal to feel downbeat on occasion, try not to let that become your new outlook on food. You should be looking forward to your next delicious keto dish! Sadly, lack of support and feelings of loneliness and inadequacy are some of the most common reasons why diets, and major lifestyle changes in general, fail.

If you have a source of negative emotions in your life, try dealing with that first, before making any dramatic dietary changes. We are emotional creatures after all, and even things that may not seem related to our dieting success can play an indirect role in shaping our motivation.

If you don't know how to infuse more positivity into your life, try doing something new. Some people like to start off their day by reflecting on a positive mantra, others prefer to engage in more social activities, travel more or pick up a light sport. Whatever you think might work for you, don't be afraid to give it a try, you have nothing to lose.

It's also important to ensure that the people in your social circle (family, friends, even your colleagues at work) understand what you're trying to achieve and have got your back. Take your time to explain your goals to them; some of them might even want to join you on this journey.

4. *Don't be afraid to ask for help*

So you've been on the keto diet for a couple of months now and you've been reading motivational books all week, but still can't shake those creeping feelings of confusion and uncertainty?

Maybe it's time to ask for help, may that be from your significant other, your best friend, or even a professional. Dieters often report experiencing feelings of shame and guilt for what they perceive as weaknesses or failures in conforming with a diet regime, and those feelings are far, far more dangerous than the setbacks that caused them.

It's okay to make mistakes and there is no shame in admitting you need assistance in reaching your goals. Don't be afraid to talk to a certified nutritionist and you might be surprised at the insight they have to offer.

5. ***Know what to expect***

If you're anxious about starting the transition to a ketogenic diet, remember that no one experience is flawless. Some people may find transitioning more difficult than others, but everyone makes mistakes and experiences setbacks at some point or another. Changing your eating habits so dramatically is no small feat, so it's wise to expect some discomfort. After all, you are asking your body to switch energy sources that, in a way, is like switching to a different kind of battery.

You may have a bit of a rocky start, feel tired often, or find it difficult to feel full after eating an entire meal. While this is normal, try not to stress your body too much. Dial back on some of the recent changes you've made, or consider new ways to substitute what you feel you've lost.

6. ***Don't neglect other aspects of your health***

While dietary changes alone can make the world of a difference in improving your overall health and weight, it's immensely helpful to just be good to yourself. Things like keeping a moderately active lifestyle, getting enough sleep, taking time off work and spending it with your family, or getting a routine physical exam, will work in tandem with your new diet to help support your health and prolong your life.

If you're struggling to incorporate more physical activity into your daily routine, think simple. Walking, cycling and other outdoor activities are not only good for your body, but also for your mind and soul. Studies are now showing that even mild exercise can have a positive impact on mental health, supporting energy levels, increasing feelings of well being and even treating depression, anxiety and stress.

7. ### *Reward yourself (but not with food)*

"I've been doing great keeping up with my diet this month, I think I should treat myself to a regular pepperoni pizza and a chocolate bar!" - Does this sound familiar? As tempting as this kind of reaction sounds, it is actually reinforcing negative ideas about your newly embraced diet.

Specifically, that it's a harrowing chore you have to put up with until the next time you can reward yourself with "normal" food. Thinking this way won't do you any good in the long run and, if you really dislike the way you are eating, you could try to improve your current diet.

That being said, it still helps to set goals and reward yourself when you achieve them, just don't do it with more food. A good way to go about it is to pamper yourself. Treat yourself to a lovely day at the spa, get a professional massage, go on a shopping spree or try an outdoor activity you've always wanted to try but never got around to.

This way, you're pumping some positive reinforcement into your life and it will make you feel better about your diet.

8. *Don't be a perfectionist*

Of all the dieting pitfalls that can stop your progress in its tracks, none is as insidiously damaging as perfectionist thinking. Whether it's counting calories, obsessing about minor setbacks or trying to assemble your dinner according to a mathematical formula, it's not sustainable to have this kind of relationship with food.

The drive for nourishment is one of out strongest instincts, so eating should still be about delighting your senses and making you feel full and satisfied. Follow the keto guidelines, but prepare the food you'd like to eat and don't be afraid to step outside your comfort zone and get inventive!

9. *Drink plenty of water*

It cannot be stressed enough how important adequate water consumption is to your overall health, your sense of fullness after a meal, your energy levels, your immunity and even the way you look. Yes, water has been shown to help maintain a youthful looking skin and prevent the formation of fine lines.

It is indispensable in virtually all-major bodily functions - it improves digestion, keeps the kidneys healthy, and promotes the formation of muscle tissue. Sadly, study after study has shown that most people don't drink nearly enough water, a situation that is particularly worrisome in children. A person's water needs can vary greatly depending on the their environment and their overall health.

If you're not sure how much you should be drinking, don't count on your thirst to tell you the amount of water you need. Instead, try drinking one small glass of water every hour or at least 8 tall glasses of water every day.

10. *Make eating healthy a lifelong goal, not a one-off project*

For most people, reaching their health and weight goal is not the most difficult aspect of dieting. Keeping that weight off and making dietary changes that last a lifetime is what's truly challenging. Reaching your primary goals can happen within months, so bear in mind from the very start that you'll eventually hit the maintenance phase.

At this phase, you're no longer trying to shed extra weight or improve your blood test results; you're just trying to preserve what you have achieved. For long-term success, it is important that you keep making small steps and gradually work towards making the ketogenic diet your normal, every day way of eating.

How to measure ketones?

Since the ketogenic diet is one that is low in carbohydrates and moderate in proteins, your body starts to train itself to use the fatty acids that are stored in the muscles to produce energy. In the process, a by – product, called ketones, is produced during the metabolic state called ketosis.

The state of ketosis helps to improve your body's sensitivity towards insulin and also helps to reduce any inflammation in the body thereby reducing the risks of any chronic illnesses. It also leads your body to have better metabolism and stronger muscles.

Setting yourself up for success: 10 tips to boost your motivation

As mentioned earlier, when your body is in the state of ketosis, it releases certain products called ketones, which can be measured to assess the effect that the diet has on your body. It is always good to keep the ketones in your body at moderate levels. Let us look at a few ways to do the same.

Measuring Your Ketones

Ketones are of three types: Acetoacetate, Beta Hydroxybutryate (BHB) and acetate. It is very easy to assess the number of each of these ketones in your body since,

1. Acetate is released through your breath

2. BHB, which is not necessarily a ketone but acts like one, is in the blood stream and is used to produce energy by the cells

3. Acetoacetate is released through the urine

You have to remember that it takes time for your body to slip into the ketosis state of metabolism, which implies that you need to identify the right time to test the levels of ketones in your body.

Blood Ketone Meter

This technique can be used to measure BHB in the blood. This method gives you the right number but is an expensive and invasive method to use. If you do not like to pierce your finger or are afraid to do so, you should steer clear of this technique.

One of the brands that you should use is the Precision Xtra blood glucose and ketone meter. It is a worthy buy but there are certain components of this tester that are hard to replace. The ketone strips used to find the count of the ketones in the body cost $4 for each strip. If you are someone who wants to perform this test every day, you may want to look for an alternative method of testing.

Breath Taking

This is a cheaper and a non – invasive technique that can be used to measure the levels of acetone in your body.

The Ketonix Acetone Breathalyzer is an inexpensive way to test the ketone levels in your body. You will however, need to remember that the ketones in your blood cannot be measured by this breathalyzer on account of the fact that the ketones in your blood are often affected by water and consumption of alcohol.

This method of testing is least expensive since you will only have to buy the Breathalyzer once and will be able to test the level of ketones in your blood whenever you want to. You will never have to draw any blood from your body either.

The LED light, when you blow into the mouth piece of this breathalyzer will glow in a certain color which will give you the right number of ketones that can be found in your breath. Let us take a look at what the colors mean:

- Blue – 0 – 150 nmol/L

- Green – 150 – 400 nmol/L

- Yellow – 400 – 930 nmol/L

- Red - >930 nmol/L

Yellow and Red are the two colors that are directly linked to nutritional ketosis.

The device is as big as a marker and has USB cord attached to the base that is 3 feet in length.

It is very easy to set up this device. All you need to do is download a small program onto your computer after which you will need to create a profile. Attach the USB port to your computer and wait for the hardware to setup before you click start. Blow into the exhale unit and wait for the LED light to glow.

Urine Ketone Strips

This is a technique that is used by many people to identify the level of ketones in their body. The strips that are used are often not accurate when it comes to understanding the level of ketones in your blood.

It is an inexpensive way to use since you will only have to spend $10 for 100 strips, which is an extremely small amount of money to spend when compared with any other method that is used. You can test yourself every single day and still avoid spending too much money.

When you start with the ketogenic diet, you will find that the strips do not show you the right number of ketones in your body. This is because your body has still not adapted to storing ketones or fats in your body. Once your body has adapted to the changes in the diet, you will be able to assess the right number of ketones in your body.

There will be a lower level of ketones in your body since your body will start to store them in the cells to produce energy. If the ketone levels that are shown have not started to decrease in number it means that you are making a mistake in your diet.

Any changes that are made to hydration will change the level of ketones in your body and also reduce their concentration in blood. If you constantly hydrate yourself, the ketone levels in your urine will be diluted thereby giving you a lower number. If you find a higher number of ketones in your body, it means that you are dehydrated.

Frequently Asked question

If you are trying the ketogenic diet for the first time, there are numerous questions that you may have. This chapter addresses some of the questions that have been asked very often about the ketogenic diet. You will be able to understand the topics that are being discussed to a good extent.

When does your body move into the metabolic state, ketosis?

When you first switch to the ketogenic diet, your body will need to adapt to the changes that are made to the diet. Your body will not move into the state of ketosis within a few hours or days. It will take a minimum of five days for your body to adapt to the changes. If you are waiting to move into the ketosis state, it is advisable to exercise on an empty stomach since you will be able to jump-start your system. However, you have to keep in mind that you consume a lot of water.

Do calories need to be counted?

The calories that you consume every day always matter. But, the intake differs from person to person depending on the age, gender and any other aspects of their health. You have to make sure that you eat properly and are never leaving your body to feed off of any stored fats or ketones on a regular basis.

Setting yourself up for success: 10 tips to boost your motivation

The most important thing you have to do is stay away from snacks. You do not have to worry too much about your caloric intake when you are on a ketogenic diet since you will be consuming a sufficient amount of proteins that will keep you full for longer periods of time.

How to track the intake of carbohydrates?

You can use different apps to track the intake of carbohydrates. You may not be able to count the calories that you consume every meal but will be able to get the estimate of the number of calories you have consumed throughout the day.

What foods am I allowed to eat?

This is a question that most people ask since they are new to the ketogenic diet. The second chapter in this book gives you a clear idea on the foods that you can and cannot eat.

Is too much fat okay?

It is all right to consume a lot of fat, but this is only if it is necessary for you. You have to remember to avoid consuming too much that you overshoot your caloric needs since you will be unable to lose weight. You will probably be wondering how you may over eat when on the ketogenic diet, but this is a very high probability. Keep a keto calculator on your phone, which will help you assess the right number of proteins, and fats that you need to consume every day.

Where can I find recipes for low carb foods?

This book contains tons of recipes that you can incorporate into your diet. You can modify the recipes to match your tastes while making sure that they still are low in carbohydrates. If you are looking for new recipes, you can use the Internet since there are so many available online.

Keto Recipes

Salads

Beefsteak & eggs salad

Serves 4

Ingredients

- 2 sirloin steaks, about 1 pound each

- 8 cups mixed greens

- 4 free range eggs, hard-boiled

- 2 Tbsp pine nuts, toasted

- 1 large garlic clove, crushed

- 2 Tbsp Dijon mustard

- 2 Tbsp fresh rosemary

- 1 Tbsp red wine vinegar

- 4 Tbsp extra virgin olive oil

- Salt & pepper to taste

Directions

1. Rub the steaks on both sides with 1 Tbsp of olive oil. Season with rosemary, salt and pepper. Let the steaks rest at room temperature for 1 hour, allowing the flavors to seep into the meat.

2. Place the eggs in a pot and cover them with water by about 1 inch. Bring them to a boil and cook over medium heat for 8 to 10 minutes, until hard. Remove them from the pot and let them cool on a wood cutting board.

3. Preheat your grill pan over high heat. Place the steaks in the pan and cook without turning for 2 and a half minutes. Turn and cook for another 2 and a half minutes. Turn the heat down to medium and cook for a few more minutes, until the steaks reach your desired doneness (about 5 minutes for rare). Transfer the steaks onto a plate and let them rest, loosely covered, for at least 10 minutes.

4. While the steaks are resting, prepare a vinaigrette in a small bowl by mixing together the vinegar, garlic, mustard, salt and pepper. Add the remaining olive oil in a thin stream, whisking continuously until emulsified.

5. Place the greens in a large salad bowl. Cut the steaks into slices about 1/2 inch thick, toss them into the bowl and mix well. Slice the eggs into quarters and arranged them over the salad mixture.

6. Top with pine nuts, drizzle with the dressing and serve right away!

Hearty Cobb salad

Serves 2

Ingredients

- 1-cup cherry tomatoes, halved
- 4 slices of ham
- 2 slices of turkey bacon
- 2 free range eggs, hard-boiled
- 2 cups romaine lettuce, coarsely chopped
- 1 avocado, diced
- 1 ounce of blue cheese
- 1 Tbsp extra virgin olive oil
- 1 Tbsp apple cider vinegar
- 1 teaspoon lemon juice
- 1 teaspoon Dijon mustard
- Salt & pepper to taste

Directions

1. Hard boil the eggs as per the method described in the previous recipe.

2. Cook the ham and turkey bacon in a non-stick skillet over low heat, flipping and turning often so that every piece fries evenly.

3. In a small bowl, prepare the dressing by whisking together the olive oil, vinegar, lemon juice, Dijon mustard, salt and pepper.

4. On a salad platter, start by distributing the roughly chopped lettuce on the bottom. You will be arranging the ingredients in tightly packed rows. Slice the eggs, cut the bacon and ham into squares, cut the tomatoes into halves and cube the avocado and the cheese. Set them in rows on top of the lettuce.

5. Spread the dressing over evenly and serve.

Nutty avocado, bacon & goats cheese salad

Serves 4

Ingredients

- 12 strips of bacon

- 2 avocados, diced

- 1 cup goat's cheese, diced

- 3 handfuls of baby spinach (about 4 ounces)

- 1/2-cup walnuts, toasted

- 3 Tbsp lemon juice

- 1/4-cup extra virgin olive oil

- 2 teaspoons Dijon mustard

- Salt & pepper

Directions

1. Preheat the over to 400°F (200°C) and line a baking dish with parchment paper. Cut the goats' cheese into 1/2-inch pieces and place it in the dish. Bake on the upper rack for a few minutes, until golden.

2. While the cheese is baking, fry the bacon in a non-stick skillet over low heat, until crispy, and then cut into bite-sized squares.

3. In a large salad bowl, place the baby spinach and add the diced avocado, fried bacon and goat's cheese and mix lightly. Roughly crush the nuts and sprinkle on top.

4. Assemble a dressing by whisking together the lemon juice, olive oil, Dijon mustard, salt and pepper. Drizzle on top and serve right away.

Luscious chicken, avocado & mozzarella salad

Serves 4

Ingredients

- 2 avocados, diced

- 1 boneless, skinless chicken breast (from roast chicken or grilled separately)

- 1 medium sized butter head lettuce

- 1-cup mozzarella, diced

- 1 medium sized red bell pepper, sliced (julienne)

- 1/2-cup sun dried tomato, finely diced

- 1 clove garlic, finely diced

- 2 Tbsp balsamic vinegar

- Salt & pepper to taste

- 2 Tbsp extra virgin olive oil (optional)

Directions

1. Roughly chop the lettuce and place it in a roomy salad bowl. Cut the chicken breast into bite-sized chunks, dice the avocados, mozzarella cheese and a few slices of sun dried tomatoes and add everything the bowl.

2. Julienne the pepper, finely dice the garlic clove and add to the mix. Drizzle balsamic vinegar on top, season with salt and pepper and mix well. Serve right away or refrigerate for later.

Thai shrimp salad

Serves 4

Ingredients

- 1 pound shrimp, peeled, deveined

- ¾ cup extra virgin olive oil, divided

- 2 teaspoons fish sauce

- 2 teaspoons sambal oelek

- 4 tablespoons soy sauce

- 1-tablespoon brown sugar (optional)

- 2 tablespoons red bell pepper (sweet or hot as per your taste), minced

- 1-cup sugar snap peas

- 8 cups romaine lettuce, shredded

- 1 cup sweet bell pepper, thinly sliced

- 1-cup cherry tomatoes, halved

- 1 bag kelp noodles, cook according to the instructions on the package

- 2 tablespoons fresh mint, chopped

- 2 tablespoons fresh cilantro, chopped

- ½ cup peanuts, roasted, crushed

- 1/3-cup fresh lime juice

- Salt to taste

- Freshly ground pepper to taste

Directions

1. To make the dressing: Add ½ cup oil, fish sauce, soy sauce, brown sugar, lime juice and minced pepper into a bowl and whisk well. Set aside.

2. Place a large skillet over medium high heat. Add 2 tablespoons oil. When the oil is heated, add half the shrimp. Sprinkle salt and pepper over it. Sear on both the sides until done. Transfer into a large bowl. Repeat with the remaining shrimp and 2 tablespoons oil.

3. Add rest of the ingredients into the bowl of shrimp and toss well. Pour dressing over it. Toss well and serve right away.

Mixed green spring salad

Serves 4

Ingredients

- 8 slices bacon, cooked until crisp, crumbled
- 8 ounces mixed greens
- 4 tablespoons Parmesan, shaved
- 6 tablespoons pine nuts, roasted
- Salt to taste
- Pepper to taste
- 8 tablespoons keto raspberry vinaigrette or to taste

For the Keto raspberry vinaigrette:

Makes ¾ cup

Ingredients

- ¼ cup white wine vinegar
- ¼ cup golden raspberries
- 15-20 drops stevia or to taste
- ¼ cup extra virgin olive oil

Directions

1. To make raspberry vinaigrette: Add all the ingredients into a blender and blend until smooth. Strain with a wire mesh strainer. Discard the seeds and retain the

liquid (vinaigrette). Use 8 tablespoons of this or as per your taste. Store the remaining in a small jar in the refrigerator.

2. Add all the ingredients of the salad bowl. Pour dressing and toss well. Serve right away.

Tomato mozzarella arugula tower

Serves 4

Ingredients

- 4 medium ripe tomatoes

- 4 cups arugula

- ½ cup fresh basil, chopped

- 4 tablespoons olive oil

- 2 tablespoons balsamic vinegar

- 6 ounces part skim mozzarella, cut into slices

- Freshly ground pepper to taste

- Salt to taste

Directions

1. Add basil, olive oil, pepper, vinegar, salt and pepper into a blender and blend until smooth. Transfer into a bowl and set aside.

2. Cut a thin slice of top and bottom of each tomato. Now slice each tomato into 3 equal thick slices. Sprinkle a pinch of salt and pepper and keep it intact (the shape of the tomato after the top and bottom was sliced)

3. Place about ¾ cup arugula over each plate. Place a tomato over the arugula in each plate. Layer with mozzarella slices followed by arugula followed by some more mozzarella.

4. Finally drizzle the dressing over it and serve.

Lobster salad

Serves 4

Ingredients

- 1 ½ pounds Northern lobster
- 4 cup Chinese cabbage (Bok-Choy or Pak-Choi), shredded
- 1 small red pepper
- 8 medium spring onions
- 2 tablespoons sesame seeds
- Salt to taste
- Pepper powder to taste

For the dressing:

- 4 tablespoons rice vinegar
- 4 tablespoons tamari sauce
- 2 tablespoons canola oil
- 2 teaspoons sesame oil
- 2 teaspoons ginger, minced

Directions

1. To make the dressing: Mix together all the ingredients of the dressing in jar and shake vigorously. Set aside for a while for the flavors to blend in.

2. Mix together rest of the ingredients in a large bowl. Pour dressing over the salad. Toss well and serve.

Soups

Roasted broccoli & cheddar soup

Serves 4

Ingredients

- 1 large broccoli, cut into florets

- 2 Tbsp extra virgin olive oil

- 1 medium onion, diced

- 3 cups broth (vegetable or chicken)

- 1-cup cream

- 2 cloves garlic, crushed

- 1 teaspoon fresh thyme, chopped

- 1 1/2 cups aged cheddar cheese, shredded

- 1 Tbsp grainy mustard

- Salt & pepper to taste

Directions

1. Preheat the oven 400°F (200°C) and line a baking dish with parchment paper. Arrange the broccoli florets in a single layer, drizzle with olive oil and season with salt and pepper. Roast until golden brown, about 20 minutes.

2. Heat 1 Tbsp of olive oil in a large pan; add the chopped onion and sauté lightly over medium heat for about 5 minutes. Add the crushed garlic and thyme, and cook until fragrant, for about a minute.

3. Add the broth and the baked broccoli, bring everything to a boil, then reduce the heat to low and allow the soup to simmer, covered, for about 20 minutes.

4. Gently whisk in the cream, mustard and cheddar cheese and add salt & pepper to taste.

5. Pour the soup into a blender and blend away until it reaches the desired consistency. Serve warm.

Cream cauliflower & bacon soup

Serves 4

Ingredients

- 1 cauliflower head, cut into florets

- 8 strips of bacon

- 1 medium onion, finely chopped

- 6 spring onions, thinly sliced

- 4 cloves garlic, crushed

- 4 cups chicken broth

- 1-cup heavy cream

- 2 bay leaves

- Salt & pepper to taste

Directions

1. Fry the bacon in a deep non-stick pot over low heat, until crisp. Put the bacon on a plate and set aside, leaving the fat in the pot.

2. Add the chopped onion, crushed garlic and half of the sliced scallions and cook slowly, stirring constantly and scraping any brown bits stuck to the bottom, until the onion is golden. Pour in the chicken stock, heavy cream and bay leaves and stir gently. Bring to a simmer, add the cauliflower, then cover the pot and let it cook slowly until the cauliflower is tender, about 25 minutes.

3. Remove the bay leaves and blend the soup in a blender or food processor, until the desired consistency is reached. If the soup is too thick, whisk in another cup of hot chicken broth. To serve, sprinkle with crisp bacon bits and the remaining scallions and season with salt and pepper.

Quick super foods soup

Serves 4

Ingredients

- 1 medium cauliflower head, cut into small florets
- 1 medium yellow onion, finely diced
- 2 garlic cloves, finely diced
- 5 ounces of arugula
- 4 handfuls of baby spinach (or 1 bag)
- 4 cups vegetable or chicken stock
- 1-cup cream
- 1/4 cup melted butter
- 1 handful fresh parsley, roughly chopped
- 1 bay leaf
- Salt & pepper to taste

Directions

1. In a large cooking pot, melt the butter over low heat, add the diced onion and garlic and cook until golden. Wash the spinach and watercress and set aside to drain.

2. Cut the cauliflower into small florets and add to the pot. Toss in the bay leaf and cook gently, mixing frequently. After about 3 minutes, add the spinach and arugula and

cook gently until the greens are softened, about 3 minutes.

3. Pour in the vegetable stock, cover the pot and let it simmer until the cauliflower is almost done. Pour in the cream and cook for another few minutes, allowing the cauliflower to cook thoroughly.

4. Season with salt and pepper. Take off the heat, remove the bay leaf and blend the soup with a hand blender until creamy. Serve with a sprinkle of parsley or refrigerate for up to 3 days.

Autumn pumpkin chipotle soup

Serves 6

Ingredients

- 2 cups pumpkin puree
- 4 cups chicken broth
- 1 medium onion, chopped
- 1 clove garlic, crushed
- 1/2-cup heavy cream
- 2 Tbsp extra virgin olive oil
- 1-teaspoon ground coriander
- 1-teaspoon ground cumin
- 2-teaspoon sugar substitute (stevia works best)
- 1 Tbsp chipotles in adobo sauce
- 2 Tbsp red wine vinegar
- 1 handful fresh cilantro, chopped (optional)
- 2 Tbsp pumpkin seeds, roasted (optional)
- Salt & pepper to taste

Directions

1. Heat the olive oil in a non-stick pan and sauté the chopped onion for a few minutes, until slightly golden. Add the chipotles and ground spices to the pan and

cook for 3 minutes to release all the fragrances. Pour the chicken broth and pumpkin puree to the mix and let it simmer for 5 minutes.

2. Take the pot off the heat and blend the soup until smooth using a hand blender. Pour in the heavy cream and red wine vinegar and return to the heat, letting everything simmer for another 5 minutes.

3. Season with salt and pepper. Serve hot, garnished with fresh cilantro and roasted pumpkin seeds.

Portuguese green soup

Serves 4

Ingredients

- ½ chicken, do not remove fat or skin
- ½ cup onions, chopped
- 1-cup sweet potato, peeled, chopped into chunks
- 1-teaspoon garlic, chopped
- Salt to taste
- Pepper to taste
- 4 -5 cups water
- 1-tablespoon coconut oil
- ¾ pound collard greens or kale, discard hard stem, chopped into 1-inch slices

Directions

1. Place a large saucepan over medium heat. Add oil. When the oil is heated, add onions and garlic and sauté until onion is golden brown. Add water and chicken. Cook until the chicken is tender. Remove with a slotted spoon and set aside on your work area.

2. Add sweet potatoes into the saucepan and cook until tender.

3. When the chicken is cool enough to handle, discard the bones, skin and fat from the chicken.

4. Add the chicken back into the saucepan. Also add greens and cook until the greens wilt.

5. Take off the heat. Season with salt and pepper and serve hot.

Chilled avocado soup

Serves 8

Ingredients

- 3 cups Hass avocado puree
- 3 cups vegetable broth
- 1-cup heavy cream (optional)
- ½ cup cilantro, chopped
- 2 jalapeno peppers, deseeded, chopped
- 2 teaspoons ground cumin
- 1 teaspoon salt or to taste

Directions

1. Add all the ingredients to a blender and blend until smooth.

2. Chill until use.

3. Serve in individual bowls.

Cream of mushroom soup

Serves 3

Ingredients

- 1 package Portobello mushrooms

- 1 medium onion, chopped into chunks

- 1 ½ teaspoons tamari

- 1-tablespoon coconut oil

- 3 cups water

- 2 teaspoons mushroom soup powder

- ½ cup whipping cream

Directions

1. Place a saucepan over medium heat. Add oil. When the oil is heated, add onions and sauté until translucent. Add mushrooms and tamari and sauté for a couple of minutes.

2. Add water and simmer for 5 minutes. Add soup powder and simmer for another 3-4 minutes.

3. Remove from heat and blend (either all of it or half of it) until smooth. Place the saucepan back on low heat. Add cream and heat for 2-3 minutes. Serve hot.

Chicken enchilada soup

Serves 6

Ingredients

- 5 stalks celery, chopped
- 3 teaspoons garlic, minced
- 9 ounces chicken, cooked, shredded
- 1 ½ cups tomatoes, chopped
- 1 large red bell pepper, chopped
- 6 cups chicken broth
- 12 ounces cream cheese
- 4 tablespoons olive oil
- 3 teaspoons ground cumin
- 1-teaspoon cayenne pepper
- 1 ½ teaspoons chili powder
- 2 teaspoons oregano
- Freshly ground pepper to taste
- Salt to taste
- Juice of a lime + extra to serve
- 1/3 cup fresh cilantro, chopped
- Sour cream to serve

Directions

1. Place a large saucepan over medium high heat. Add oil. When the oil is heated, add garlic, bell pepper and celery and sauté until celery is lightly soft.

2. Add tomatoes, salt and pepper and cook until the tomatoes are soft. Add cumin, chili powder, cayenne pepper and oregano and sauté for a minute. Add broth and cilantro and mix.

3. Lower heat and simmer for 15-20 minutes. Add chicken, lemon juice and cream cheese and simmer for 10 minutes.

4. Serve in bowls. Drizzle some lemon juice and sour cream and serve right away.

Roasted garlic soup

Serves 3

Ingredients

- 1 whole bulb garlic
- 2 shallots, chopped
- 3 cups cauliflower, chopped
- 2 teaspoons extra virgin olive oil, divided
- Freshly ground pepper to taste
- 1/2 teaspoon salt or to taste
- 3 cups vegetable broth

Directions

1. Preheat the oven to 400°F (200°C).

2. Discard the outermost layers of the garlic bulb. Keep the bulb whole. Do not separate the cloves. Slice ¼ inch from the top of the bulb.

3. Place the garlic bulb on an aluminum foil sheet. Brush with ½ teaspoon oil. Wrap the bulb.

4. Place the garlic in the oven and roast for about 30-35 minutes. Cool for a while. Unwrap and squeeze the pulp from each garlic clove.

5. Place a saucepan over medium heat. Add remaining oil. When the oil is heated, add shallots and sauté until light brown.

6. Add the garlic pulp and rest of the ingredients. Cover with a lid. Bring to the boil.

7. Lower heat and simmer until tender. Blend the contents in a blender or with an immersion blender until smooth.

8. Taste and adjust the seasoning if necessary. Heat thoroughly.

9. Serve in bowls.

Main Dishes

Hamburger patties in creamy marinade

Serves 4

Ingredients

For the patties:

- 1 1/2 lbs. beef, ground (choose pieces that have a bit more fat)

- 1 large free-range egg

- 1/3-cup feta cheese

- 4 Tbsp fresh parsley, finely chopped

- 1 clove garlic, crushed

- 1 Tbsp extra virgin olive oil

- 1 Tbsp butter

- Salt & pepper to taste

For the marinade:

- 3/4-cup heavy whipping cream

- 4 Tbsp fresh parsley, chopped

- 3 ripe tomatoes, finely diced

- 1 yellow onion, finely diced

- 1 Tbsp tomato sauce

- Salt & pepper to taste

Directions

1. Place the hamburger ingredients in a bowl and mix well, using your hands. Form 8 to 10 burger shaped patties.

2. Heat the olive oil and butter in a non-stick pan and fry the patties until they start to turn golden. Cover the pan for a few minutes if necessary.

3. Dice the onion, add it to the pan and cook until translucent, about 3 minutes. Dice the tomatoes as fine as you can. When the patties are almost done, add the diced tomatoes, tomato sauce and cream, and stir well. Allow everything to simmer for about 10 more minutes.

4. Add salt and pepper to taste and serve with parsley sprinkled on top.

Eggplant & beef pizza

Serves 4

Ingredients

- 2 large eggplants
- 3/4 lb. beef, ground
- 1/2-cup chunky tomato sauce
- 2 cloves garlic, crushed
- 1 small red onion, finely chopped
- 1 1/2 cups shredded mozzarella cheese
- 1-teaspoon basil & oregano mix
- 1/4-cup extra virgin olive oil
- Salt & pepper to taste

Directions

1. Preheat the oven to 400°F (200°C). Slice the eggplants in about 1/3 inch thick slices, coat with olive oil. Line an oven tray with parchment and bake the eggplants for about 20 minutes.

2. In a saucepan, heat up 2 Tbsp olive oil and gently cook the diced onion and crushed garlic over low heat, until fragrant. Add the meat and fry until the meat has turned a nice color. Pour the tomato sauce in next, add salt and pepper and let it simmer for about 15 minutes.

3. Remove the eggplant tray from the oven and spread the meat and tomato mixture evenly over the eggplants. Top with shredded cheese and the herb mix. Return the tray to the oven for another 10 minutes, until the cheese has melted and the pizza has become a light golden-brown color.

4. Serve right away!

Greek style chicken pesto casserole

Serves 4

Ingredients

- 1 1/2 lbs. boneless, skinless chicken thighs
- 1/2 cup red pesto
- 1 1/2 cups heavy whipping cream
- 1/2 cup pitted olives, green & black
- 1/2 lb. feta cheese, diced
- 1 garlic clove, crushed
- 1 Tbsp butter
- Salt & pepper to taste

Directions

1. Preheat the oven to 400°F (200°C). Cut the chicken thighs into smaller chunks, season with salt and pepper. Melt the butter in a non-stick pan over low heat and fry the chicken until golden, about 10 minutes.

2. In a small bowl, mix the pesto and whipped cream. Toss the fried chicken in a baking dish and add the pitted olives, diced feta cheese and crushed garlic. Spread the pesto and cream mix evenly on top. Bake the casserole for about 30 minutes until it has turned a nice golden-brown color. Serve warm and refrigerate the leftovers.

Mediterranean baked fish & veggies

Serves 4

Ingredients

- 2 1/2 lbs. white fish fillet (cod or hake)
- 1 leek, chopped
- 1 medium yellow onion, thinly sliced
- 2 sweet kapia peppers, sliced
- 3 plum tomatoes, chopped
- 1 fennel, chopped
- 1 small carrot, sliced
- 1/2 cup pitted kalamata olives, halved
- 1/2-teaspoon fresh parsley chopped
- 1/2 teaspoon fresh thyme, chopped
- 1 lime, thinly sliced
- 1/2 cup white whine
- 3 Tbsp extra virgin olive oil
- 1/2-cup butter, softened
- Salt & pepper to taste

Directions

1. Preheat the oven to 400°F (200°C). Line a baking dish with a piece of aluminum foil, making sure it is large enough to fold over and seal the dish in.

2. Cut the fish fillet into smaller chunks and toss them into the dish. Slice and chop all the vegetables as instructed and disperse them evenly on top and around the fish.

3. Drizzle olive oil on top, and add the butter in small dollops. Add all the herbs and spices.

4. Fold the foil and seal it carefully. You can also add another piece of foil on top, and secure it at the corners.

5. Bake for 30 to 40 minutes and serve hot.

Coconut shrimp and avocados

Serves 2

Ingredients

- 1 avocado, peeled, pitted, chop into bite sized cubes

- 2 cups shrimp

- 2 teaspoons Sriracha sauce or any other hot sauce

- 1-tablespoon natural peanut butter

- 2 teaspoons shredded coconut

- 2 tablespoons light coconut milk

- Cooking spray

Directions

1. Place a nonstick pan over medium heat. Spray with cooking spray. Add coconut milk, peanut butter and hot sauce. Stir until well combined.

2. Add shrimp and cook until shrimp are tender. Remove from heat and sprinkle coconut over it.

3. Place avocados on a serving plate. Place the shrimp over it and serve.

Steak with mushroom port sauce

Serves 4

Ingredients

- 1 pound rib eye steak

- 5-ounce mushrooms

- 1-ounce heavy cream

- 2-ounce port wine

- 1/2-tablespoon butter

- Salt to taste

- Pepper to taste

Directions

1. Season the steak with salt and pepper on both the sides.

2. Place a cast iron skillet without a handle on high. Add butter and steak and cook until brown on both sides.

3. Then place in the oven and bake in a preheated oven at 450° F until cooked. Flip sides half way through baking.

4. Remove and cover with foil. Keep aside.

5. In the same skillet, add port wine, mushrooms and cream. Place on medium flame and cook until the sauce thickens.

6. Pour over the steak and serve hot.

Zucchini casserole

Serves 6

Ingredients

- 12 cups zucchini, diced

- 1 red bell pepper chopped

- 1 yellow bell pepper, chopped

- 1-cup quinoa, cook according to the package instructions

- 1 1/2 cups cheddar cheese, shredded

- ¾ cup olive oil

- 1 1/2 teaspoons dried basil

- 3 eggs, beaten

- Salt to taste

- Pepper powder to taste

Directions

1. Mix together all the ingredients in a bowl. Transfer to a greased baking dish. Spread all over the dish.

2. Bake in a preheated oven at 350° F until top is golden brown.

Low carb pad Thai

Serves 4

Ingredients

- 1/2-bag kelp noodles
- 1 small white onion
- 2 cloves garlic, peeled
- 4 tablespoons natural peanut butter
- 2 tablespoons soy sauce or tamari or liquid aminos
- 1-teaspoon red pepper flakes
- 2 tablespoons lime juice
- 1-tablespoon sesame seeds, toasted
- 2 tablespoons scallions, chopped
- 2 tablespoons cilantro, chopped
- Salt to taste
- Pepper powder to taste

Directions

1. Add kelp noodles to a bowl of water and soak for a while.

2. Blend together in a blender, peanut butter, onion, tamari, lime juice, garlic, pepper flakes, pepper, and salt until smooth and creamy.

3. Drain the noodles and place in a large bowl. Pour the peanut butter mixture over it and toss well.

4. Sprinkle sesame seeds and cilantro and serve.

Roasted red pepper and garlic stuffed mozzarella chicken

Serves 4

Ingredients

- 4 chicken breasts, boneless, skinless

- 4 tablespoons extra virgin olive oil

- 20 fresh basil leaves

- 12 cloves garlic

- 2 tablespoons all purpose chicken seasoning

- 16 small herb marinated mozzarella balls (you can also use normal ones if these are unavailable)

- 2 roasted pepper, halved lengthwise

- 2 tablespoons fresh oregano, chopped or 1 tablespoon Italian seasoning

- Freshly ground pepper to taste

- 1 teaspoon garlic salt or to taste

Directions

1. Using a meat mallet, pound the chicken slightly and butterfly it. Stuff the basil leaves and garlic in each of the chicken breasts.

2. Place 4 mozzarella balls over each. Place a red pepper halve over the balls (1 halve per chicken breast). Sprinkle the oil that is present in the marinated

mozzarella over the chicken breasts if desired. Also sprinkle the olive oil over it.

3. Sprinkle garlic salt and pepper generously. Finally sprinkle oregano over it. Place in a lined baking dish.

4. Bake in a preheated oven at 400° F up to 40 until tender.

Spicy sausage & cabbage skillet melt

Serves 6

Ingredients

- 6 links spicy Italian chicken sausages, discard casings, chopped

- 2 1/2 cups purple cabbage, shredded

- 2 1/2 cups green cabbage, shredded

- 1 large onion, chopped

- 3 slices Colby Jack cheese

- 3 tablespoons coconut oil

- 3 tablespoons fresh cilantro, chopped

Directions

1. Place a large skillet over medium high heat. Add oil. When the oil is melted, add onion and cabbage and sauté until tender.

2. Add sausages and sauté for 7-8 minutes. Remove from heat and set aside for 5 minutes.

3. Place cheese slices on top and cover. Set aside for 5 minutes. Uncover and stir.

4. Garnish with cilantro and serve right away.

Desserts

Caramel macchiato cheesecakes

Serves 9

Ingredients

<u>For the cheesecakes:</u>

- 1-cup cream cheese

- 2 Tbsp melted butter

- 3 large eggs

- 3 Tbsp espresso powder

- 4 Tbsp sugar substitute (stevia is best)

- 1 Tbsp sugar-free caramel syrup

<u>For the frosting:</u>

- 1-cup mascarpone cheese

- 3 Tbsp soft butter

- 3 Tbsp sugar free caramel syrup

- 2 Tbsp sugar substitute (stevia)

<u>Extra:</u>

- 1 Tbsp soft butter to grease the cupcake molds

- 1 Tbsp instant coffee for decoration

Directions

1. To prepare the cakes, preheat the oven to 350°F (180°C). Place all the cheesecake ingredients in a blender and blend until smooth. Pour the mixture into a cupcake tin lined with paper molds, or pour it into 9 greased individual cupcake molds. Bake for 15 minutes until firm, remove from the oven and let them cool in the freezer for 1 hour or in the refrigerator for at least 3 hours.

2. For the frosting, whisk the butter, caramel syrup and sweetener to a fluffy consistency. Add the mascarpone and in whisk in gently, until smooth.

3. To serve, pipe the frosting onto the cheesecakes and lightly sprinkle instant coffee on top.

Peanut butter chocolate fudge

Serves 6

Ingredients

<u>*For the fudge:*</u>

- 1/2-cup peanut butter

- 1/2 cup softened coconut oil

- 1/4 cup almond milk

- Vanilla extract to taste (1 teaspoon or less)

- 2 teaspoons stevia or preferred sugar substitute

<u>For the chocolate topping:</u>

- 1/4 cup cocoa powder

- 2 Tbsp coconut oil

- 2 Tbsp stevia or preferred sugar substitute

Directions

1. Melt the peanut butter and coconut milk together in a pot over low heat. Pour in a blender and add all the other fudge ingredients. Pulse until smooth.

2. Line a small loaf pan with parchment and pour the mixture in. Refrigerate for a few hours, until set.

3. For the sauce, whisk all the ingredients together to obtain a thick topping and drizzle over the fudge once it has set completely.

4. Serve chilled and keep refrigerated for up to 4 days.

Easy flourless brownie

Serves 12

Ingredients

- 6 free-range eggs

- 3/4 cup melted butter

- 1/3 cup cocoa powder

- 1-teaspoon vanilla extract

- 1/2-teaspoon baking powder

- 2/3-cup cream cheese

- 3 Tbsp stevia or preferred sugar substitute

Directions

1. Preheat the oven to 350°F (180°C). Toss all the ingredients in a tall bowl and, using a hand blender, pulse until smooth.

2. Line a baking dish with parchment and pour the mixture in. Bake for 20 to 25 minutes, until cooked all the way through.

3. Allow the brownie to cool completely, and then slice into thick squares and serve.

Mint and chocolate chip ice bombs

Serves 7

Ingredients

- 1/2 cup full fat mascarpone cheese or creamed coconut milk

- 1 ounce 90 % dark chocolate, chopped

- 2 1/2 tablespoons powdered erythritol or Swerve or to taste

- Liquid stevia drops to taste (optional)

- 1/2 teaspoon peppermint extract or 3 teaspoons fresh mint, minced

Directions

1. Add all the ingredients to a blender and blend until smooth. Transfer into a bowl.

2. Add about 2 tablespoons of the mixture into round molds or small silicone muffin molds.

3. Freeze until set. Remove from the molds and serve.

Blueberry cheesecake popsicles

Serves 5

Ingredients

- 1-cup cream cheese

- 4 cups fresh blueberries

- 6 tablespoons erythritol or Sweetener or to taste

- 4 cups heavy whipped cream.

Directions

1. Add all the ingredients except cream into a blender and blend until smooth.

2. Transfer into a bowl. Add cream and fold gently.

3. Pour into Popsicle molds and freeze until done.

4. Remove the molds from the freezer 10 minutes before serving. Invert on to a plate and serve.

5. Alternately, you can pour in the ice cube trays and freeze.

6. You can replace blueberries with any other berries of your choice to get a new flavor. You can also use mixed berries.

Cream cheese clouds

Serves 12

Ingredients

- 1/4-cup butter, unsalted, softened

- 4 ounces cream cheese, softened

- 1/4-teaspoon vanilla extract

- 1/4-cup granular splenda or erythritol

Directions

1. Add cream and splenda to the mixing bowl and beat with an electric mixer until firm peaks are formed.

2. Line a baking sheet with wax paper. Drop spoonfuls cream on the baking sheet.

3. Chill and serve later.

Vanilla crème pudding parfaits

Serves 8

Ingredients

- 2 cans (14.5 ounces each) full fat coconut milk, chilled
- 2 teaspoons vanilla extract
- 20 drops liquid stevia
- 1/2-cup walnuts, chopped
- 1 1/2 cups fresh berries of your choice (blueberries/blackberries/strawberries/ raspberries etc.
- Ground cinnamon to garnish

Directions

1. To make vanilla crème: Pour coconut milk to the bowl of your stand mixer. Add stevia and vanilla extract. Whisk until well combined.

2. Add berries and walnuts to a bowl. Toss well.

3. Take 8 parfait glasses. Add about 3 spoonfuls of vanilla crème into each of the glasses.

4. Use about 1/2 the berry mixture and layer over the vanilla crème. Spoon some vanilla crème in each glass. Next divide and place the berry mixture. Place about a teaspoon of vanilla crème on top.

5. Sprinkle ground cinnamon over it.

6. Chill and serve.

Cinnamon coconut peanut butter cookies

Serves 8

- 2 eggs

- 2 cups peanut butter

- 1/2 cup butter

- 1/4 cup shredded coconut

- 1 cup erythritol

- 2 tablespoons ground cinnamon

- A pinch salt

- 1 teaspoon vanilla extract

Directions

1. Add peanut butter, butter, eggs and erythritol into a mixing bowl and beat well with an electric mixer. Add cinnamon, salt and coconut and fold to form dough.

2. Divide into balls and shape into cookies. Place the cookies on a lined baking sheet. Leave a gap of at least an inch between 2 cookies. Press the cookies with a fork.

3. Sprinkle coconut and bake in a preheated oven at 350°F (180°C) for about 15 minutes.

4. Remove from oven and place on a wire rack. Cool completely.

5. Serve. Store unused ones in an airtight container.

Before You Go

If you liked this book, you may like these other popular books from **Jennifer Sullivan**

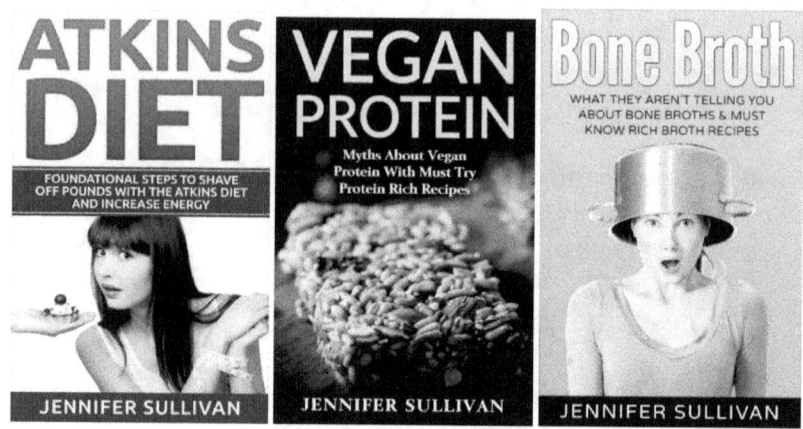

Check out more books from **Jennifer Sullivan**

Visit Below!

https://www.amazon.com/Jennifer-Sullivan/e/B01J4O3N6U/

If you didn't download your **FREE** Gift to *"Habits: The Essential Guide"* yet you can get it by visiting the link below.

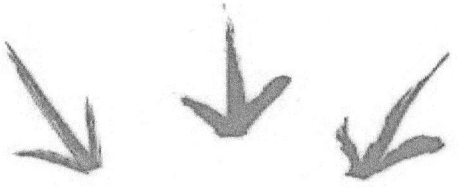

https://cueballpublishing.leadpages.co/free-habits-ebook/

Conclusion

Thank you again for joining me on this journey!

I hope this book was able to help you learn more about the ketogenic diet amidst all of the common confusion.

The next step is to implement these strategies to lose weight and feel great!

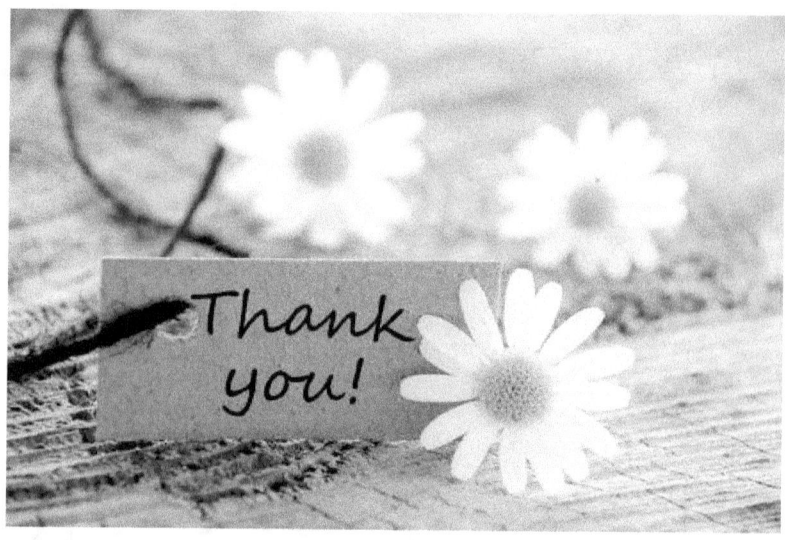

Finally, if you enjoyed this book, then I'd like to ask you for a favor, would you be kind enough to leave a review for this book on Amazon? It'd be greatly appreciated!

Thank you and good luck!

www.ingramcontent.com/pod-product-compliance
Lightning Source LLC
Chambersburg PA
CBHW062052280526
45788CB00003B/1199